Armor of Faith

Armor of Faith

A MOTHER'S MEMOIR

Viviane M. Philmon, Ed.D.

ISBN-13: 9781523960262
ISBN-10: 1523960264
Library of Congress Control Number: 2016902631
CreateSpace Independent Publishing Platform
North Charleston, South Carolina

To: KII & J.C.

The wait is over

Acknowledgements

THIS MANUSCRIPT, ARMOR OF FAITH …A mother's memoir, has taught me a lot about myself. I am ever evolving. My journey thus far substantiates the fact that life is full of twists, twirls and unexpected turns. I'm learning to trust my inner- voice which beckons me to delve deeper, to go higher, to expand my consciousness and to embrace my experience of FAITH on a more personal level day by day.

In the spirit of utmost gratitude, I take this opportunity to express my love and appreciation to all who contributed to the completion of this project.

My family: Nobody has a more caring and supportive family of parents, siblings, children, cousins, aunts, uncles, nieces and nephews… NOBODY!

My proof readers: Janice Melton, E. Christine Henry, Barbara Johnson, Tara Johnson, Tamika Lee, Tiffaine Stephens, Jaime Gage, Breana Goodall-Fleming, William Savage, Shelly Casey, Zenobia Chisholm, and Brianna Tranby.

My photographer, graphic artist, adopted sons, co-workers, sorors, forever friends, prayer warriors: Ronica Martin, Ben Kepley, Jarrett

Cagle, Christopher Hicks, Aaron Cummings, Julian Mayo, Alex Ozojie, Staff members of Postlethwait Middle School, Mrs. Susan Whitaker, Mrs. Retha Organ (*I'll never forget how you stood in the gap for me!*), Dr. Robin Smith, Xio Axelrod, Denise Hicks-Barnes, Delphine Henry, Debra Reid, Frank Johnson, James and Ava Perrine, Joey Cohen, Dolly Washington, Rabbi Elliot Holin, The members of High Street Church of God, Mrs. Virginia Washington, Mrs. Louisetta James, The members of Crossroad Christian Church, Marcia Cagle, Geneva Goldsboro, Kim Brown, Beulah Yarborough, Pete & Susan Cook, Elaine Van Huis, Lisa Orlando, Barbara Atwell, Michael Williams, …and many, many others far too numerous to mention and far too precious to neglect.

To God be ALL GLORY AND PRAISE !!!

Contents

Prologue

THIS IS A LOVE STORY. It is a tale of fear and faith; hurt and healing; triumph and tragedy. A saga of this nature has been more than difficult to write because of the emotional pain associated with it. While clearly the healing process has begun, scars are also evident. I am now certain that the true essence of this account can be fully expressed at this time of essential restoration.

The majority of this publication is centered on the time that began in the Spring of 2002. During that period, my children were ages twelve, nine, and eight.

Even now, as I sit at my computer, I marvel over the realization of the events that have occurred over the past fourteen years. *"WOW!"* is often spoken from my lips as I reflect on this difficult time. Sometimes, it feels as if I'm looking at someone else's life. The truth of the matter is that I wish there was another more adequate individual to bear this burden. There have been times when I have uttered, "Why me?" I now bask in the notion that I was elected to fulfill such an awesome assignment.

This project came to fruition largely because of my personal journals. I have utilized journals for many years and began to journal when I was married. I found it to be a comfort to me throughout problematic periods of my married life. I have included actual journal entries for you to read in this work because I feel they provide insight into my life at that time in a way that narrative recollections cannot. The journal entries are dated, bolded, and italicized. You will notice that they are **not** all in chronological order. This was done intentionally as a means to express how chaotic my life was during that worrisome period. The facts presented are also compilations of documentation, recollections, and notes from doctor's visits.

My heart's desire at this time is to share what I've learned in an effort to enlighten and assist another family who may be facing a similar health-related dilemma. I have verbalized on many occasions that I'm looking forward to the day when an individual comes to me and shares that he or she has experienced a miracle because of the insight gained from applying what was learned in this book. On that great day, I will smile and exhale with a renewed sense of satisfaction knowing this voyage was designated for a purpose extending beyond my family.

Throughout this book, you will sometimes read the words, "my husband" or the name, "Ed". In 2002, the man referred to was indeed my husband. The educator in me is reminded of the fact that "ed" is the suffix that means, "in the past". It is imperative that I acknowledge his input during that difficult time. Although we are no longer married, I would be remiss in not mentioning his presence and tumultuous silence. I now realize that his ability to distance himself emotionally was a coping mechanism during critical phases of his life. During our acrimonious divorce, I learned he had been secretly reading my journals throughout our marriage. Therefore, he is largely responsible for convincing me that my writing was worth reading. (*Thanks, Ed!*) I now bless him and pray for his peace.

My oldest child, my son Edwin, can be described as handsome, friendly, muscular, comical, and introspective. Sometimes I affectionately refer to him as my Chocolate Prince. The term is fitting not only because of his smooth, dark skin, but also his confident demeanor and love of chocolate. When he was in elementary school,

I sometimes teased him by calling him a "chocoholic" because of his fondness for dark, sweet treats. Edwin has been known as the prankster of the family and would often perform harmless practical jokes to get a laugh. Even as a child, I noticed that he attempted to make situations lighter when life became too intense or serious.

My second child, my daughter Ebony, is a slender, adorable, sweet girl with beautiful honey-colored skin and long, thick hair. In a crisis situation, she appears to internalize her true feelings. As the middle child, I sense that she desires balance and stability. She is a child who is cooperative and obedient. At times, I will find her alone in her room reading a book or involved in an activity that has her attention, and she is focused and quiet. Although most people comment that she looks like her father, she reminds me of myself. I, too, am the middle child, and am most comfortable in a calm and tranquil environment.

My youngest child, my daughter Imani, is a drama queen. From the very beginning, this pretty little one has clearly understood her role as the baby of the family. She sometimes behaves in an overbearing manner in order to have her way. Yet on the other hand, Imani has a kind, generous, spirit. I often tell people she is my most affectionate child. There are times when she will walk up to me while I'm cooking dinner or am engaged in some other household chore and wrap her arms around me to give me a warm squeeze. Then, she'll look directly at me, smile, and walk away without saying a word. Whenever I gaze into her beautiful, brown eyes, it becomes apparent that she is a compassionate individual. Imani is the type of child who is free enough to cry during a movie (one of her favorites is Warner Brothers' My Dog Skip). I have often stated that, "Imani will give you her last." Imani seems to understand the true principle of giving. Somehow, she knows, "The more you give, the more you get."

I believe Imani was sent to earth as a gift from God to teach me a valuable lesson about Faith. Incidentally, Imani is the Kiswahili name, which translated means, "My Faith". At the time of her birth, I had no idea that naming her Imani would be so significant for the intensive journey I would face in an effort to save her precious left arm.

Some people believe miracles originate in heaven. I have recently learned that miracles come from deep within. If you believe in miracles, this book is a MUST READ! If you are a skeptic or a pessimist, I strongly challenge you to read as well. If you are somewhere in-between, I trust that you will allow your curiosity to propel you towards the pages of this book. I welcome you all and I am confident that the events that unfold on the pages of this book will impact your life with great significance.

The title of this book is **Armor of Faith…**A Mother's Memoir. I trust you will be encouraged as you read the following pages. More importantly, if you are facing a similar situation with your child or a loved one, I hope and pray you will realize that you too are equipped to confront your oppressive test. A friend recently told me, "A test makes a testament." As I give honor and glory to God, here is my testament.

Blessings,

Viviane

Put on the whole armor of God, that you may be able to stand against the wiles of the devil. For we do not wrestle against flesh and blood, but against principalities, against powers, against the rulers of the darkness of this age, against spiritual hosts of wickedness in the heavenly places. Therefore take up the whole armor of God, that you may be able to withstand in the evil day, and having done all, to stand.

(Ephesians 6:11-13)

❖ All scripture references are from the New King James Version of the Holy Bible.

O N E

2002

⁓

__March 2002__
__It's difficult to write now...so much is happening!__

DISNEY WORLD IS THE PLACE where dreams come true. However, for me it was the beginning of a horrific nightmare. It was March 26, 2002. During Spring Break, our family went to Disney World for the first time. The weather was absolutely beautiful! The temperature was 75-85 degrees daily. It was truly a welcome change from the chilly atmosphere of Dover, Delaware. Mickey, Minnie, Donald, Daisy, Goofy, and the rest of the Disney characters made the trip all the more meaningful as we immersed ourselves in the sights, sounds, and smells of the Animal Kingdom Lodge.

One evening, while I was preparing bath water for my eight-year old daughter, Imani, I noticed an odd-looking lump on the upper segment of her left arm. I gently touched it and asked her if it hurt. She simply replied, "No, Mom." The lump was small and soft to the touch, yet it was noticeable as it protruded slightly through her skin. Immediately, I thought it could have come from a rough-house activity with her older brother, Edwin. Being four years older than Imani, there were times when he'd wrestle with his sister and I would cringe thinking he may be too rough with her.

After her bath, I again examined the peculiar looking lump on Imani's arm. This time, I asked her father to check it out. He studied her arm for awhile and then stated, "We'll have to take her to see a doctor when we get back home." His response satisfied me for the moment. However, something in my spirit left me feeling terribly unsettled. From that point on, the mysterious lump hovered in the back of my mind. I checked it several times a day for the remainder of our trip.

A few weeks passed before we were able to get an appointment to be seen by a local physician once we returned home. During that time, the lump grew and changed in consistency. While the top of it felt soft and spongy, the base was becoming more compact and firm. With each daily arm examination, countless thoughts gallivanted through my mind as if they were being lead by a team of wild horses.

I believe most parents would agree that one child in every family seems more accident prone than the others. Among my own siblings, it was my sister, Chrissy. As a child, I can remember numerous trips to the emergency room due to some injury of Chrissy's. There was the time when she was six or seven years old and pushed broken pieces of crayons into her nose. The pieces were so far up in her nostrils that my father and mother were unable to retrieve them with their fingers. My father finally had to use tweezers to get the broken crayons out. Another time, as a young teenager, she became light-headed and almost fainted when she got so frustrated about having a congested nose while suffering from an upper respiratory infection, that she blew her nose too hard and broke some blood vessels. I'll never forget seeing my panic-stricken father rushing to her as the blood spurted from her nose like a fountain. He caught her in his arms just before she collapsed onto the floor and took her to the emergency room. The doctors stuffed her nasal cavities with gauze for two or three days. There were countless episodes of falling over chairs, regularly dropping and breaking glasses during family dinners, tripping on stairs, and so on. My mother jokingly started referring to my second eldest sister as, "Calamity Chris".

Considering my three children, I'd have to say that Imani seems the most prone to mishaps. She is my "Calamity Chris". When Imani was three years old, she developed an extremely high fever just before Thanksgiving Day. At one point, she was so hot that the blood vessels in her eyes burst, leaving the whites of her eyes completely bloodshot. To make matters worse, her entire little body was covered with hives when she woke up the day after Thanksgiving. We rushed her to the hospital and she was diagnosed with a condition called Kawasaki Syndrome, which is a rare disorder usually found in Asian or Caucasian boys. The pediatric specialist strongly encouraged us to allow our daughter's body to be intravenously pumped with gamma globulin, which is plasma donated in human blood, in order to rebuild her immune system.

After several grueling days in the hospital, we were finally permitted to go home with a recovering Imani. She was given a prescription for chewable aspirin to be taken once daily. We were told to keep a close watch over her. Through further research, it was found that some children who have been diagnosed with that particular syndrome often develop heart problems. The aspirin was proposed as a preventive measure to offset any potential problems with her heart.

On another occasion, Imani fell and fractured her left elbow at the tender age of four. She was playing outside with her siblings and the two family dogs. As usual, big brother Edwin presented his little sisters with a challenge. Instead of swinging on the toy set like most children, he decided it would be a good idea to test his two sisters' physical prowess by demonstrating how to grasp the top bar of the apparatus with both hands and gingerly maneuvering his movements in order to get to the other side (*Imagine an activity similar to military basic training*). Edwin performed the task with the ease of a trapeze artist. He then coerced his two sisters to follow his lead.

Ebony is a tomboy at heart and thus succeeded with the challenge. When it came to her brother, Ebony would readily accept most challenges and complete them effortlessly. Imani's turn took much verbal prompting from both of her siblings. As the youngest of the three, Imani often appeared to seek validation from her older siblings. She bravely grasped the top bar of the swing set with all of her might, but along the way, she lost her grip and fell to the ground. The result was a fractured elbow. Her little, neon pink cast is tucked away in my bedroom chest as a reminder of that frightful incident.

An additional event involved Imani suffering second-degree burns on her right arm. All of the children were home from school because of a teacher in-service training session that I was required to attend at my school. When I went to work that morning, I was secure in leaving the children home with their father. I later learned that my three children were left home alone to fend for themselves. Around lunchtime, the school secretary alerted me to the phone with an urgent message. She said, "Viviane, call home. There's an emergency with your children." I immediately called home and heard Ebony's quivering voice reporting, "Mom, Imani is burned badly. Please come quick!"

I rushed home to find Imani's right arm burned so severely that the pinkish-white flesh beneath the surface was evident. Imani had been preparing to make a cup of hot chocolate in the microwave oven. When the microwave chime alerted her that the water was ready for the chocolate mixture, Imani attempted to lift the mug full of hot water from the microwave oven to the kitchen countertop. While in transit, the blistering moisture from the mug spilled onto Imani's right arm and the scalding water caused first and second degree burns!!

The emergency treatment consisted of a special burn cream and gauze dressings that had to be changed three times daily.

As I reflect back on those days of attending to the burns on Imani's right arm, it is clear to me now that the focus on her right arm is directly related to my attention to Imani's left arm in sunny Florida during our Disney World vacation. It was time to get ready for a pilgrimage involving Imani's left arm that would forever change our lives.

T W O

Cancer ??

❖ *Cancer (n). A malignant tumor that invades healthy tissue and spreads to other areas.*

FROM THE END OF APRIL to late May 2002, I felt like a caged hamster running around on a wheel. I was in the midst of completing coursework towards my Master's Degree in Curriculum and Instruction. My graduation date was scheduled for May 19, 2002. I was required to complete a major project as well as what seemed like tons of paperwork. The children were busy with school and extracurricular activities. I attempted to focus on my marriage, my growing children, my housework duties, and teaching responsibilities…the daily grind. That combination at times was overwhelming. On top of everything else, there was that weird looking growth on Imani's arm. To my dismay, every time I examined it, I had to admit that it appeared a bit larger.

I often tell people that I took a crash course in cancer the summer of 2002. Before then, I wasn't aware that there are so many different types of cancers. I was also unaware of the legion of statistics relating to cancer. For example, I have since learned…

* Eating lots of fruits and vegetables can help reduce your cancer risk.
* Adequate nutrition may benefit a child with cancer by maximizing quality of life.

❖ Webster's Classic Reference Library (New Revised Edition)

* Some cancers cause no physical pain at all.
* Alternative treatments for cancer have been proven to be not useful or even harmful, but are still promoted as cures.
* The state of Delaware ranks fourth in the nation in overall cancer rates.
* Delaware is the first state in the nation to guarantee health insurance for each person diagnosed with cancer.
* Cancer is the leading cause of death for children in the United States.
* Within the next decade, cancer may become the leading cause of death in the United States.
* Nationally, dramatic survival improvements have been achieved in patients diagnosed with cancer at age fifteen or younger.
* More than 90% of patients live at least five years after their cancer is diagnosed. This five-year survival mark is the point at which a patient is considered "cured" since the tumors rarely occur later.

My husband was employed at Dover Air Force Base in Dover, Delaware. Therefore, the first doctor we saw was a military physician who referred us to a local dermatologist. The skin specialist scratched his chin and looked over his wire-rimmed glasses with deep concern.

Viviane M. Philmon, Ed.D.

He suggested we go to a well-known children's hospital located in the northeastern region of the country, so we could be close to family members in the event that hospitalization became a necessity.

That's when I became painfully aware of the procedures involved in the medical field. It was pure agony. I became familiar with THE GAME.

The phone calls, the automated voice prompts, **the waiting**, the referrals, the doctors' busy schedules, **the waiting**, the appointments, the sometimes insensitive receptionist, **the waiting**, the crowded waiting rooms, the short time you actually get to spend with the doctor, the unanswered questions, **the waiting**, the irritating, frustrating **WAITING GAME!!!**

By and by, we met the Chief Orthopedic Surgeon of the children's hospital, who will be henceforth referred to as, Dr. Portalmen*. He presented himself as a charming, tall, lanky white-haired man with a gentle demeanor. After examining Imani, he suggested that we schedule her for a biopsy in order to better determine what was going on with her left arm.

With the biopsy scheduled just four days prior to my graduation date, my emotions became hopelessly tangled. I distinctly remember breaking down hysterically as I witnessed the hospital staff wheel Imani away on a gurney to the operating room. As the automatic doors closed between us, Ed stood by me stoically, engaged in light-hearted conversation with a friendly nurse.

During the surgery, we were told to wait in the family lounging area. It was a large room with a television, magazines, a snack machine, and anxious family members. Once in a while, a doctor or nurse would come into the waiting area to update parents on the progress. I witnessed lots of hugging, tears of joy, clapping, and sighs of relief. Being a private person, I can remember thinking, *"Wouldn't it be better to share news of this nature with families in a more intimate setting?"*

---

* Name changed to protect his identity.

8

After what seemed like an eternity, a nurse summoned Ed and me to another smaller, secluded room. *"Good,"* I thought. *"We're receiving VIP treatment today."* I felt as if someone had been reading my mind. Shortly, Dr. Portalmen appeared and told us Imani was in the recovery room and that all was well. He also said the mass was of a strange gelatinous nature with many fibers.

He confirmed that the base of it was curiously more firm than the rest of the mass and that we would be contacted after he received the lab results.

As our confidential session continued, I recall Dr. Portalmen saying his professional experiences up to that point led him to believe that the strange mass could possibly be a rare cancer but that he was going to remain optimistic and hope for the best. In the moments that followed, I almost blacked out. It felt as if the room slowly began to spin and I was about to fall flat onto the floor even though I was sitting down. My stomach began to do obnoxious twists and turns and left me feeling like I was going to regurgitate! I could hear Dr. Portalmen talking, but I suddenly imagined the words slowly pouring from his lips as a dark, thick molasses. My heart began to beat so fast that I could hear thumping inside of my ears! I glanced over at Ed to see if he was being affected in the same way I was and I wondered, *"Is this doctor talking about our child?"* Ed sat still and intently listened as Dr. Portalmen explained further. Looking back, I am convinced that this was Dr. Portalmen's way of attempting to caution us for the detestable road that lay ahead.

My spirit became even heavier as I left the room that day. How could I think about the possibility of a child of mine with cancer? I'd spent so many years striving to live a health-conscious life! Furthermore, my marriage was falling apart, the 2002 school year was quickly ending, and my other children needed me just as much as Imani. My inner Being screamed,"How am I supposed to function with so much pandemonium in my life?"

T H R E E

Myxofibro Sarcoma

June 19, 2002
Dr. Portalmen called today to tell me he wants to do another surgery. Imani's arm is really large (swelling). He confided that he believes it to be a rare form of cancer. I don't want to believe it is cancer! This is really getting to me. I'm sooooooo tired!!!

THE DAY I GOT THE call from the hospital that confirmed a diagnosis of cancer will forever be etched into my memory.

I was preparing a meal for the children when the telephone rang. Dr. Portalmen was on the other end of the line. In a composed manner, he shared news about the pathology report. I grabbed a nearby notepad and responded with, "Can you please spell that?" Dr. Portalmen offered, "M-Y-X-O-F-I-B-R-O-S-A-R-C-O-M-A." My eyes filled with tears and my hands shook uncontrollably as I scribbled the letters on the scrap paper. Dr. Portalmen alleged that the recommendation for this rare type of cancer was amputation. He stated the cancer was believed to be low-grade (I/III) and wanted to speak with me and my husband to discuss a plan for an additional surgery.

When I hung up the phone, I felt as if I were in the Twilight Zone. I knew the children were nearby playing gleefully, but I sensed I had suddenly stepped outside of my "self". My five senses all became dull. The "ME" I thought I knew became a vapor. My comprehension was totally disrupted. I couldn't seem to wrap my mind around the fact that I had just been told my child had cancer! ***"OH MY GOD!!!"*** My thoughts were in a disheveled state. A million theories sprinted through my mind.

I finally regained my composure enough to call Ed. After dropping the bomb, there was an uneasy soundlessness. At long last, Ed spoke, "We need a second opinion." "Yes!" I chimed in. I began to feel ecstatic about the idea of exploring another option. The doctors at this hospital had to be making a mistake. We would go elsewhere to get more information. The news we were given had to be completely inaccurate!

I spent the remainder of that day in shock. There were phone calls made to family members and close friends. I remember lots of gasping and crying. I recall gentle words of encouragement. Most of all, in a desperate state of confusion, I recollect gazing at my dear, sweet Imani.

F O U R

Sugar-Coating

July 8, 2002
A friend came by to have prayer with me today. She
embraced me and whispered in my ear, "Trust me. The joy
is coming." That embrace and those kind words worked
wonders for me! I feel comforted by the Holy Spirit. She
also told me to read Psalm 23 and Psalm 119.

IT WAS A CHILLY DAY in June when we met Dr. Wolfe*. Although
it was a typical summer day, there was definitely an eerie chill in
the atmosphere on that day. The Chief Orthopedic Surgeon had
scheduled a meeting with our family in order for us to talk with
someone else at the children's hospital regarding their decision
to amputate Imani's left arm. While the doctors at the hospital
encouraged us in our quest for another opinion, it was clear that
they wanted to waste no time in moving forward with the surgery.
Therefore, the doctors decided to introduce us to Dr. Wolfe, a
sarcoma specialist.

---

* *Name changed to protect his identity.*

Following a brief physical examination of Imani's arm, Dr. Portalmen shared a little about his colleague who was called upon to impart his professional judgment on the matter at hand. As we waited, Imani needed to use the bathroom, so I figured I would accompany her since the initial exam was over and the Specialist had not yet arrived.

After Imani and I exited the restroom, we held hands and headed back to our previous location. As we got closer to the door, I heard a *"tick-tick-ticking"* sound from a machine. The noise prompted me to look towards a door on my left. The door to the room was ajar and I saw a man squatting by a machine as a facsimile was being transmitted. He held several pages in his hand as more papers were discharged from the facsimile machine. *"Hmmm?"* I thought.

A few minutes passed after Imani and I re-entered the examination room. Then, the "Specialist" came in who was introduced as Dr. Wolfe. Coincidentally, he was the same individual I had briefly glanced at moments prior. Dr. Wolfe held a stack of papers in his hand that I am certain could only have been scrutinized briefly. Dr. Wolfe was a fifty-something Caucasian man with a stern expression and indifferent demeanor. He barely smiled and offered no words of encouragement on Imani's behalf. Dr. Wolfe gave Imani a quick once-over then prodded her into the waiting area where she could play with toys.

I was taken aback by this man's brusque manner. As a physician dealing with a child and obviously overwhelmed parents, I would certainly have imagined someone more sensitive and compassionate. Once Imani left the room, Dr. Wolfe looked at Ed and me and stated very matter-of-factly, "Look, I'm not gonna sugar-coat this for you ... **You have to amputate that arm!**" Instantaneously, I was both shocked and insulted. His words stung like a slap in the face. I grew indignant. After all, this man knew nothing about my child!

I supposed that he did not do a thorough enough evaluation of the facts. Suspecting he had just received Imani's records (or some sort of information relating to our case), Dr. Wolfe was egregious in his technique and I resented everything about him. He concluded his delivery with a warning to us as parents to have Imani placed on the surgery schedule "ASAP." He further cautioned that there was no alternative to the amputation! I left the hospital that day filled with anguish and wept quietly all the way home.

> ### <u>June 29, 2002</u>
> *I'm in a scary place! Two doctors have told us that Imani's left arm must be amputated!!! I'm numb … I'm terrified. This is grueling! I can't believe I'm in this place. I've been praying for a MIRACLE! Ed and I are on A+ behavior towards each other. I can tell he's as scared as I am. I feel like there is NO WAY I can justify allowing the doctors to amputate her arm. She's such a loving child with wonderful hugs. God – I need your guidance. Help me to truly believe in your healing power.*

FIVE

The Second Opinion

THE TASK OF GETTING A second opinion for Imani's unpromising diagnosis was completely laborious. Time was not on our side as Imani's left arm swelled daily. Family members and close friends graciously offered suggestions about contacting institutions that specialized in cancer treatments. Even with the overwhelming gestures of love and support, it was a fearful time. Our search for a second opinion lead us to Maryland, New York, Pennsylvania, Georgia, and finally to Tennessee.

With each hopeful encounter, we were faced with more disappointment and despair. We were directed to send the original MRI* report along with paraffin slides from the biopsy report to each establishment we contacted for assistance. The procedure further involved telephone calls to doctors for referrals and an endless paper trail pursuit. Again, the waiting period was physically and emotionally exhausting.

Along the way, I gained a wealth of information about medical doctors. I have since learned that it is imperative to play an active role in healthcare procedures and treatment plans. Many individuals go to the doctor and blindly do whatever the medical professional tells them to do because the doctor is trained to know more than we are about

---

* MRI= Magnetic Resonance Imaging

our bodies. Not so! I have come to the realization that each individual case needs to be viewed in isolation. Unfortunately, for many reasons, doctors are often unable to spend the necessary time getting to know each patient in an intimate manner. My family needed to get to the root of our child's problem. We needed a health care professional who was committed to assisting us in our quest for Imani's optimal health and wellness. We required healing for our daughter – not a quick-fix.

We forged onward throughout those critical days. All the while, the medical team called our home to strongly encourage us to place Imani's name on the surgery schedule for the removal of her left arm. One conversation I distinctly remember took place between me and Dr. Portalmen. He began by telling me he was on vacation and gave me his home telephone number so that I could have direct access to him. I was impressed by what came across as concern for Imani.

Dr. Portalmen began to describe how the operation he planned to perform was such an "aggressive surgery" and that it would take all day to complete the procedure. Immediately, I imagined Dr. Portalmen cutting through my child's flesh and bones with an instrument resembling a chainsaw. I became ill and grief-stricken. He further cautioned me about a concern that the growth on Imani's arm could metastasize to other parts of her body including her chest and lungs. I told Dr. Portalmen that I was **not** ready to make the decision to amputate Imani's left arm. The doctor's tone became a bit more unyielding. He insisted, "I don't think you realize that we are trying to save your daughter's life." I forced out the following words while fighting back tears, "I do understand what you're saying but, **I can't agree to it!**" I hung up the telephone and barely made it to my bedroom before I broke down with irrepressible sobs.

Another physician in Maryland was kind and amiable while giving us some hope. During our visit, he shared that he would contact a colleague to see if there was any more that could be done with Imani's swollen arm. By that time, Imani's left arm had grown so much in size that it was noticeably larger than the right arm. When she wore T-shirts, her expanding arm made the clothing appear to be ill-fitting. Imani was embarrassed to wear summer tops like her sister. I winced inside as I observed her shrinking back self-consciously and holding her body in a manner that signified insecurity and low self-esteem.

Time mandated our wait through the weekend before we could get the follow-up information from the doctor in Maryland. That weekend, every minute felt like an hour, and each hour like an eternity in hell! The first thing Monday morning, I made the call to the doctor in Maryland. His voice was cautious and courteous. An explosion erupted in my head as the doctor explained how he would not be able to remove the mass on Imani's arm because the cancer resembled a gelatinous-fibrous type of matter that is very rare. He concluded with a tender apology and concurred with the decision to amputate Imani's arm. In that moment, helplessness and hurt traded places with hope.

July 11, 2002
I'm concerned about Imani. I'm concerned for all of my children. Following our visit to the hospital in Baltimore for a second opinion, Imani stated, "I thought you said I didn't have cancer." (I could have died a thousand deaths!) She also voiced her concerns with, "When will this swelling go away?" and "I don't want another surgery!" and "When can I stop going to the doctor?" and "I want this to be over." I'm at a loss for words ... I don't have the answers.

Next, we made contact with a well-known cancer center in New York City. However, the doctor we were referred to was out of the country attending a medical convention. We were told he would not be returning for two weeks. With that in mind, I decided to leave the doctor an urgent telephone message with the hope that he would call upon his return to the United States. When the doctor did call back, he was abrasive and rude in his tone towards me. He bellowed, "Weren't you told you needed to amputate the arm?" I was unprepared for his insincerity. He ended our discussion with, "Don't bother bringing your child here!" Again, I sobbed uncontrollably at the conclusion of that appalling phone call.

I also made contact with a good friend of mine in Georgia who is a pediatrician. She gave me the names of several hematology oncologists she knew in Philadelphia, Pennsylvania. After a few days, she called me back and sweetly relayed, "I'm so sorry, Viviane. I wish I could be of more help."

Still another place of contact was a world-renowned center in Tennessee. I found the staff there to be compassionate during our telephone exchanges. They too wanted us to send all medical records, x-rays, paraffin slides, and other documentation before they would offer a definite answer that would warrant a trip south. We prepared and sent the appropriate paperwork to Tennessee and waited. Weeks later, an obliging physician called to share his findings. He explained that based on the test results, he believed it, "Looked like a cancer." He continued by saying that he felt the need to support the original diagnosis, but reiterated that it was very difficult to be sure because the myxofibro sarcoma is such a rare form of cancer. The medical humanitarian wished us well and discouraged us from making the trip to Tennessee.

The aching in my heart begged, *"Why doesn't each hospital do its own testing?"* I feel individual testing is especially necessary in cases where medical findings are rare. In the end, it was evident that each facility simply agreed with the original diagnosis. Therefore, the second opinion was NOT really a second opinion. In our case, the second opinion was simply the first opinion with a stamp of approval from fellow physicians.

July 7, 2002

Today I am weary. The swelling has been increasing. How could God give us such a precious gift and then have us ponder losing it? The biggest problem for me is… Once the arm is gone, there's NO turning back! How do we tell Imani we were afraid and confused during this time? How do we make a decision that is in her best interest? I'm so tired – I'm so scared!!!

Other great fears are:

1   *How do we explain this to Imani and her siblings?*
2   *What if they remove her arm and then tell us the procedure was unnecessary due to the "thing" spreading to other parts of her body?*
3   *Since Imani is feeling fine and her left arm is not giving her any discomfort, will she hate me for the rest of her life as she reflects back on these days?*
4   *What if we lose her anyway?*
5   *FEAR is not from God so, right now I must be the most ungodly person on the planet!*
6   *When will we make it to that "all right" place everyone is telling me things are gonna be?*

SIX

A Friend Indeed

July 18, 2002
Mornings are especially hard for me. I'm suffering with anxiety attacks each morning (hot sweats, heart palpitations, upset stomach). My soul aches to the core every day that I wake up to see my beautiful eight year-old with that huge lump/mass on her left arm! My mind is flooded with exasperating thoughts. Waiting for responses (a second or third opinion) from the other hospitals is painful. There's so much to do in this effort to save Imani's arm. We ALL need to be saved! Mornings are so hard for me!!

LYNN IS THE TYPE OF friend anyone would feel blessed to have. We met at Sunday school when I was 12 years-old and she was 11 years-old. I remember being intrigued by her from our first encounter. She was different. She wasn't in attendance every Sunday like my family was, but when she did attend, she always made her presence known. Lynn wasn't afraid to ask our Sunday School Teacher the tough questions I'm certain others of us were thinking. She'd blurt out things like, "How do you know Jesus looked like that?" or, "Is the Red Sea really red?" Some of the other girls disliked her, but for some reason, Lynn and I became fast friends.

As the years progressed, we grew closer. By the time we were in high school, our friendship became more solid. We shared clothes, adventures, likes, and dislikes, and we vowed to take some of our life experiences to the grave.

While attending a local college, I began to spend a lot of time at her house because my school was located close to her home and because Lynn's parents were so kind to me. They made me feel comfortable to share in family meals. I slept there often, and on occasion even did my laundry at their house. After a while, Lynn's family became an extended family for me. When she got married, I was one of her bridesmaids. Likewise, when I got married four months later, Lynn returned the favor and served as one of my bridesmaids.

Lynn's generous nature is one of the things that has kept us close over the years. She has become a wonderful resource to me. She is the type of individual who sincerely loves to give. Lynn is dedicated to helping people achieve their personal best. She chose to study religion and psychology for her profession which allows her to express herself lovingly as she assists others in managing their lives.

I clearly remember the Sunday morning that I spoke on the telephone with Lynn as she called to check on Imani. In desperation, I explained the doctor's intention to remove Imani's entire left arm. I rambled on and on about the details involving the doctor's medical findings regarding this rare form of cancer and the dangers of it spreading to Imani's chest cavity. Lynn listened intently. She allowed me to cry and vent for quite a while. Then she spoke slowly and deliberately in an effort to calm my soul. Lynn told me she had a friend who lived in Boston, Massachusetts. Her name was Lovey* and she

---

* Name changed to protect her identity

had been diagnosed with a serious blood disease, a rare cancer, that affected her lymph nodes. Lynn further shared that Lovey had met with a Japanese healer in New York City and that the man was instrumental in saving her life.

At that time, there had been many family members and friends calling our house on a daily basis to offer support and suggestions for Imani's condition. Needless to say, on that day, I was not in the mood to make another call to a stranger and possibly have my hopes crumble due to information leading to another dead end. Lynn could sense the hesitancy in my voice. Finally, she implored, "You should call Lovey. You have nothing to lose but an arm." That's what did it for me.

<u>July 19, 2002</u>

I feel totally fatigued. Mentally, Physically, Emotionally, Spiritually ... I'm approaching the point of exhaustion. I need to rest. I desire a place of refuge. My reality is too Raw! My inner core aches! Oh Lord, deliver us from this trial. I'd deliver myself if I only knew how. How? When? Why? What? What in this world is going to happen next? What's next? Where are we going with this? When can I get a break? I soooooooo need a breakthrough!

SEVEN

"If it weren't for the rocks in its bed, the stream would have no song." – Carl Perkins

SHORTLY AFTER SPEAKING WITH LYNN, I decided to call her friend Lovey. Because of Lovey's easy-going temperament, our initial conversation flowed freely. Lovey told me she had been diagnosed with a rare type of lymphoma that had manifested as a tumor in her chest. It had grown to be about the size of an orange. The doctors had given her less than six months to live and her family had prepared funeral arrangements. Lovey had received chemotherapy and radiation treatments that had taken a toll on her body.

However, she was fortunate enough to meet a man by the name of Henry Honest*. She testified with a most noteworthy assuredness, "He literally saved my life." Lovey then offered me the necessary information to contact her Japanese mentor. I readily admit that I was a bit apprehensive at that time. This was largely attributed to the fact that I was emotionally destabilized. I thanked Lovey for her openness and warmth in sharing her fascinating story with me. Before we ended our phone conversation, I asked, "By the way, Lovey, how long have you known Henry Honest?" Her answer is what prompted me to

---

* Name changed per Healer's request

dial the number to the Natural Remedies Center in New York City. "I've known him for twenty years" she affirmed.

<u>*July 3, 2002*</u>
I'm terrified! Yesterday, Ed told me that a (nosey) neighbor told him we could be arrested if we refuse to allow the hospital to amputate Imani's left arm. God Help us! That same neighbor said something about a court order and "life or limb". My mind is in a state of frenzy – I can't eat – I'm not sleeping well! God – where are you? I need help right NOW!!!

E I G H T

"At the moment of commitment, the universe will conspire to assist you." – Virginia Satir

I WILL NEVER FORGET THE day I first called Henry Honest. It was a moist and muggy day in July of 2002. The children played outside with the dogs while Ed was at work on the military base. I nervously dialed the number I was given not knowing what to expect. A meek-sounding, pleasant, female answered with a warm greeting in broken English. I asked to speak with Henry Honest hoping that I would possibly get the opportunity to talk with him within two or three days. She replied, "One moment please." *"What?"* I thought to myself, *"I know she's not actually going to allow me to speak with him right now."* Following a brief moment, a steady, practical voice spoke, "This is Henry Honest. What can I do for you?"

My frantic conversation at that juncture must have portrayed me to be the most spastic person in the universe. I heard myself rambling on and on about Imani and her grim diagnosis. I divulged information about her condition unsure of whether he wanted to hear it or not. Before I burst into tears, he interrupted me with, "Bring her to me right now." "Right now?" I managed to blurt out. "Yes," he replied. I continued with, "But my husband is at work and I live in Dover, Delaware!" The gentle voice at the other end of the line beckoned, "Then you must bring her to me tomorrow."

The family trip to New York City the following day included my father, Ed, and our three children. The excitement and anticipation was truly overwhelming. My mind was literally in a state of frenzy. When we reached our destination, I felt as if I was in a trance. The sights and sounds of New York were electric and buzzing all around me. However, I was uneasy as we approached the large apartment building which housed the Natural Remedies Center.

Seven feet of black iron doors with glass lead to the entrance of the vestibule. Once inside, we were "buzzed" past the doors and entered into a long hallway with a mosaic style tiled floor. At the end of the hallway, there was a small elevator to the left. It was painted pea green and had an eye-level, glass circular insert. The elevator doors opened in an accordion fashion that reminded me of an old movie. A small sign on the inside of the elevator instructed us to press "B" as our expedition continued downward.

Peculiarity filled the small enclosure as we reached our basement destination. The elevator creaked and jerked as the door slid open. Immediately, my sense of smell became engaged. The aroma of cedar incense, sassafras, comfrey, lemon grass, alfalfa, and a host of potent natural herbs wafted through the atmosphere and filled my nostrils. As we turned to the right, another doorway led us to where we had to make use of the buzzer system one final time. At last, we were granted authorization to enter.

Warm earth tones decorated the waiting room area. We made ourselves comfortable on the soft cream colored leather sectional chairs. Individuals of Asian descent scurried about busying themselves with various duties. Patrons waited patiently at a nearby counter as their personal prescriptions were filled from numerous large, clear jars of natural herbs. The room reminded me of a science laboratory. The walls were filled with packets of literature. Also, there were pictures of celebrities boasting testimonials from past experiences involving the center. The peaceful space was further accented with bamboo plants and lilies. Yet another outstanding feature was the Angels. There were Angels everywhere. Illustrious statues of Angels were on the coffee table. Cherubs were strategically propped over the doorways and Angelic figurines were mounted above the bookshelves. The room was filled with the presence of beautiful Angels!!!

In the midst of all the movement was a Japanese man dressed in plain clothes. Ed leaned close to me and whispered, "I'll bet that's him." We often played a game which involved guessing the physical characteristics of individuals before actually meeting them. We would later engage in whimsical conversations after our first face-to-face encounter. In this case, I shook my head in disagreement. The "Healer" I was expecting to meet would be wearing a white lab coat, an important, shiny-looking name tag and a countenance that exuded superiority. However, nothing was further from the truth.

At precisely eleven o'clock (the time of our scheduled appointment), the same diligent little man came over and introduced himself. He wore dark, loose-fitting sweat pants, a t-shirt, and flip-flops. "Which one is Imani?" he questioned while peering at both girls. "This is Imani," I responded. Immediately, he focused all of his attention on his newest patient. "May I have permission to touch you?" he respectfully asked. Imani acquiesced shyly. Then the Master Healer went to work. He removed his footwear and lowered himself to his knees in front of our daughter. As he gently touched her left arm with both of his hands, he closed his eyes and bowed his head. His breathing became intentionally loud. I was in awe of his modus operandi. The degree of reverence he exhibited towards Imani's body was absolutely breathtaking. I felt enlightened as I looked over at Imani to check on her. Imani sat still as she viewed the top of the remarkable Healer's head. She appeared to instinctively absorb all that was happening to her.

After what seemed like 3-5 minutes, Henry Honest opened his eyes, smiled at Imani, and asserted, "Do <u>not</u> remove her arm." I instantly felt as if I had won the lottery! I was elated as I fought back tears of joy! I had so many questions; *What should we do next? What should we tell the doctors? How can we get rid of that thing on Imani's arm? How did this horrible thing happen to us? When can we come back for another visit?* Henry Honest explained to us that Imani had a virus which caused some type of blockage in her meridian system. Her left arm was swelling as a result of the break-down in her body's system. He affirmed that removing her arm would not get to the root of the problem.

We were now faced with the task of detoxifying her precious body and strengthening her delicate immune system. Henry told us to change her diet completely. Imani would now have to eat more whole foods, drink lots of water and increase her intake of organic fruits and vegetables. As he spoke, I took notes and received answers to all of my queries. Finally, Henry Honest told us that Imani would have to drink a special tea, designed specifically for her, and take lots of supplements in an effort to aide in the healing process. As the assistants filled brown paper bags with ingredients for the tea, I noticed that some of the objects resembled twigs, tree bark, roots, and even corn husks. I investigated by asking, "This looks like the stuff I see when I am shucking corn." Henry smiled and stated, "That's exactly what it is." I further questioned, "What are all of these other things called?" Henry Honest simply responded with, "If I told you what it is called, you still wouldn't know what it is." I was then given a note with instructions on the proper preparation for the Japanese Tea. We left the center with a shopping bag full of ingredients for the teas and supplements.

Immediately, I decided it was best for our entire family to revamp our way of eating. If a healthier diet was good for Imani, then it stood to reason that a family diet change would benefit all of us. I decided on an "all for one and one for all" campaign.

Our vehicle on the ride home that day felt to me like a chariot supported by clouds. The next few days found me on the telephone with family members and close friends relaying what happened in New York City. One of my cousins cautiously asked me, "What makes you think this man is right when so many doctors from well-known institutions are telling you to remove Imani's arm?" To be candid, I needed a doctor with a semblance of credibility to declare something contrary to what the others were saying. My desolation caused me to step out on faith. My faith pushed me to exercise my belief that the teas, supplements, and diet change would make a positive difference in Imani's life. The Bible says, "Faith without works is dead." (James 2:26)

I decided to go to work.

July 25, 2002

Two days ago, we traveled to New York City to meet a HEALER. He is a Japanese man who really gets to the root of problems. He laid his hands on Imani and told us she does NOT have cancer! I believe him! The truth of the matter is, I want to believe something other than what the doctors are saying! The Healer also told us that Imani is beautiful, powerful and has the ability to heal herself. He gave us a bag of supplies (tea, pills, etc.) and assured us that we will see results in ninety (90) days. He also promised that we would see some "change" in three (3) days!!! WOW! The entire experience in New York was wonderful.

I had a dream last night that swelling on my left arm completely disappeared before my eyes!! It was so amazing and beautiful to see. I believe it was God telling me that Imani's left arm is going to be fine.

NINE

The Work

THE WORK NECESSARY FOR THIS exodus would prove to be painstaking. Invigorated by the elixir of hope, I knew it would take a miracle to turn things around for Imani. So, I prayed continuously for that miracle.

Getting Imani to drink the tea was not easy. Henry Honest forewarned us about the pungent taste of the tea. However, none of us were prepared for how extremely overpowering the tea actually was. The daily drama involving the tea took its toll on everyone. Sometimes, I relied on my mother or one of my sisters to talk on the telephone with Imani to get her to consume one-half cup of the prescribed tea. Other times, Imani's siblings and I cheered her on as she drank the bitter potion through a straw. Imani alleged that the taste was not as bad whenever she drank it with a straw, so I made sure there were plenty of colorful drinking straws on hand.

Sample of Imani's daily menu-1
Breakfast:
Green grapes, raisin bagel, Noni juice, water, 8 various supplements
Lunch:
Cucumbers, raw broccoli & cabbage mixed with flax seed oil, water
8 various supplements

Dinner:
Vegetable soup with brown rice, garden salad, green grapes, water, homemade juice from my juicer, 10 various supplements
½ cup of Japanese tea one hour after dinner

As time progressed, I told Imani she had to finish drinking the tea within 30-45 minutes. There were times when the one-half cup of tea ordeal lasted more than two hours. I set the kitchen timer and placed one or two dollars on the table in front of Imani as an incentive. I promised Imani that she could have the money if she finished drinking the tea before the timer rang. Rarely did this tactic work. On some occasions, Imani acted as if she did not care about the money. We tried all kinds of antics to encourage Imani to drink her tea. Some days were better than others.

Sample of Imani's daily menu-2
Breakfast:
Apples cut-up, Sun Butter, organic bread, water, Noni juice, 8 various supplements
Lunch:
Red potatoes cut-up, string beans, brown rice, grapes, water, 8 various supplements
Dinner:
Lima beans, couscous, spinach, cabbage, apples cut-up, water,
10 various supplements
½ cup of Japanese tea one hour after dinner

On the days Imani was not up for the tea, it was an incredible annoyance. My heart went out to her because I knew the tea was repulsive! Many times, I took small sips of the tea to encourage her. Day after day, month after month, things went on in this manner. Ed would often suddenly claim he had something important to do outside of our home during "tea time". Then he would disappear for hours. There were many times I thought about running away myself. However, my heart compelled me to stay, stand, and fight on.

I knew drinking the tea was imperative, so I tried sweetening it with raw honey or fruit juice. Even with the additives, Imani complained about the tea and often cried while being coerced to drink it. I suffered great difficulty while attempting to explain to her why she had to drink the tea every day. To make matters worse, Imani had to take numerous pills throughout the day. The daily routine became more and more arduous. Some days, NOTHING we tried could convince Imani to drink the appalling beverage without a battle.

Sample of Imani's daily menu-3

Breakfast:
Nectarine, oatmeal, homemade juice, water, 8 various supplements
Lunch:
Garden salad, applesauce, millet, brussel sprouts, water, 8 various supplements
Dinner:
Plum, corn on cob, broccoli, black-eyed peas with quinoa, water, 10 various supplements
½ cup of Japanese tea one hour after dinner

During that time, I busied myself with creating healthy recipes with organic foods (see Recipe section). The majority of my daily routine included listening to inspirational music and becoming inundated with reading material on optimal health and healing of the body. I enrolled Imani in ballet and yoga classes. I held the notion that pairing exercise with healthy eating would prove to be advantageous.

Furthermore, I had the task of preparing the Japanese teas and organizing the supplements. There were so many different pills that had to be taken in various combinations at different times of the day. It was all extremely rigorous and time consuming. So, I constructed a chart and displayed it in the kitchen for the purpose of developing accurate records and a visual representation of Imani's daily progress (weekly arm measurements, diet, weight gain, etc.).

Prayers and fasting became more regular activities. Family, friends, and church members alike became advocates in ways that are impossible to express. I could often actually *feel* the prayers that were dispensed on our behalf.

One local church rendered a special prayer and "laying on of hands" (2Timothy 1:6-7) by a charismatic Evangelist. Another church we visited during that time invited the five of us to a secluded room for an exceptional prayer while the Mother of the church bestowed upon Imani a prayer cloth as she explained the significance of the ritual found in the Bible (Acts 19:12). Still another minister in our area visited our home one Sunday evening for prayer with Imani. He anointed Imani with holy oil and fervently prayed with us to save Imani's left arm (James 5:14).

Additionally, I created a web page via a wonderful site (www.caringbridge.com) to share Imani's progress for well-wishers who desired weekly updates. Love poured in from cyberspace. Many people sent messages to Imani encouraging her to be strong. There were even strangers who visited our site with genuine care and concern. One kind visitor, a Rabbi, transmitted several memos as he promised to remain in prayer for Imani. I was deeply humbled by the tremendous displays of love and compassion.

<u>*July 26, 2002*</u>
Day three – Oh My God!!! We witnessed a miracle today! The large balloon-like mass on Imani's left arm has changed dramatically! Previously, it was located on the topside of her arm. It had also been hard and practically bulged through her skin. Today, it looks like a water balloon that is hanging under her little arm! There are still some parts that are hard but for the most part, the large mass is loose and hanging on the underside of her arm! The teas and supplements are really working! The prayers are working!! I can actually feel loved ones praying for us. So much is happening. I'm so relieved and happy to clearly see the change!

TEN

The Switch

_⌒_

**August 6, 2002**
**I hate the smell of hospitals. The disinfectant scent filling**
**the long corridors always upsets my stomach.**

IMANI WAS SCHEDULED FOR ANOTHER MRI and CAT* scan appointment at the hospital. My mother and Ebony accompanied us for that particular visit. Imani and her sister were born sixteen months apart, and when we're in public, strangers often ask if they're twins. Both girls usually chuckle and continue with the activity that previously held their attention. On that day, they were dressed in identical beige overall shorts outfits with matching bright t-shirts and socks. Imani wore a pink t-shirt with pink socks, Ebony wore an orange t-shirt with orange socks. Both girls had their hair intricately braided in corn-rowed styles with colorful beads that enhanced their natural beauty. White canvas sneakers gave the girls a well-groomed accent for summer.

Typically, there was a long wait to see the doctor. For example, it wasn't uncommon for us to sit and wait for one hour before the doctor appeared. Needless to say, it was extremely frustrating given

---

* CAT= Computed Axial Tomography

the reason for our visits. The girls were pleasant and playful as usual. They kept themselves busy with hand games (clapping, singing, and snapping fingers while tagging each other's hands). Their laughter and giddy exchanges proved to be a balm of comfort for my spirit.

When the receptionist finally called Imani's name, I immediately sensed that my eight-year old child was nervous. A nurse told us he needed to record Imani's weight. Then, the nurse said he needed to take Imani downstairs for the MRI and CAT scan. Again, Imani appeared hesitant. When I asked her if she was alright, she told me she needed to use the restroom. At that point, I sent both girls to the restroom as we used the buddy system for all public restroom visits to ensure their safety.

While the girls were gone, a doctor came to ask me a series of questions regarding Imani's left arm. I shared information about Imani's weekly arm measurements, diet, weight gain, changes in her behavior, and so forth. When the subject of the Healer surfaced, the physician seemed to be disinclined. She told me we should be very leery about Eastern practices because of the high levels of lead that are sometimes found in the supplements and herbal teas. The doctor informed us that Japanese medicines are satisfactory to use in an effort to prevent certain illnesses, but continued by pitiably sharing, "If cancer is already present, there is no use for the Japanese teas or supplements. There is NO CURE for cancer. The only treatments for cancer are surgery, chemotherapy, and radiation." Her sharp words offended me to no end. A waylaid feeling began to consume me. I thought, *"Does this woman realize that she is speaking about my child? This other option has got to work for us!"*

Once the girls returned, Imani had a sheepish grin on her face. Ebony seemed to be harboring some type of secret. As a mother of three very active children, this type of behavior is all too familiar. I'm used to the grins and unexplained giggle episodes.

Shortly, the nurse turned to tell us it was time for Imani's MRI and CAT scan. The nurse walked over to **Ebony** and gently took her by the hand to lead her to the testing area. For a brief moment, I stared at my mother. Everyone was silent. Imani looked like a cat that had just swallowed a canary. Suddenly, I realized what had happened: *the girls switched clothes while they were in the restroom!* Imani was now wearing the orange t-shirt and orange socks while Ebony was wearing the pink t-shirt and pink socks. The nurse had no idea that he was about to test the wrong child! I alerted him to the fact that he had taken Ebony by the hand instead of Imani. He took a second look at the girl whose hand he was holding and we all nervously laughed as Imani and I then prepared to proceed with the medical escort. Once released, Ebony went to sit with her grandmother. As I glanced over my shoulder, Ebony shrugged and stated, "Imani told me to do it."

When we arrived at the testing site, I stared intently at Imani and asked, "Why did you do that?" Imani shared that she wanted to be sure the doctors found nothing wrong with her left arm during the examinations, so she had devised a plan to outwit the doctors and have Ebony's arm assessed instead. I pulled her close to me as she climbed onto my lap. At that moment, it was clear to me that my baby was worn down. We embraced in that cold room as I rocked her from side to side. Warm tears began to fill my eyes and slowly rolled down my face. I discerned in that instance, "*Imani gives great hugs. She needs both arms in order to hug like this.*" Then I heard my child express her deepest desire, "I just want to be normal," she whispered.

ELEVEN

Accu-power

August 26, 2002
Each time we visit Henry Honest, I feel renewed and
hopeful. On the other hand, whenever we visit the other
institutions, I feel disappointed and defeated. Imani is
such a powerful force. She is a very affectionate child.
Last evening, she sat down close to me and began to rub
my feet and legs as we watched television. For the past
two nights, she's been sleeping next to me. Throughout
the day, she hugs and kisses me. Sometimes, she grabs
my face and stares into my eyes. I sense she was sent to
earth to get my attention. My Spirit is telling me to be
patient. I believe this to be part of a Divine Plan. The
prayer on my lips each day is for Strength, Courage,
and Wisdom.

IT WAS OUR SECOND VISIT to New York City to see Henry Honest.
Over the previous 11 days, our family had experienced dramatic
changes in our diets. For example, Henry Honest recommended that
Imani refrain from the following foods: dairy products, white sugar,
white flour, soy products, all processed foods, all food with dyes and

preservatives, and all meats. Instead, he encouraged us to give Imani lots of the following: water, fresh raw fruits and vegetables, and whole grains. I decided if a new diet was good for Imani, it had to benefit all of us. I did not want Imani to feel that she was being punished or singled out for a condition over which she had no control. Furthermore, I didn't want to have to prepare separate meals for my husband, myself, and my other two children and have to watch as Imani suffered in silence with separate servings of food.

During that second visit, Henry Honest stated that Imani was 32% better. I took notes as the Master Healer rendered the following from his examination; *"Large intestine – better; lungs are good; stomach – good; spleen – good; triple heaters – fine; heart constrictor – fine; small intestine - much better; heart - Beautiful!; gall bladder – good; liver - very good; bladder – good; kidney - a bit tired due to detoxification; hormones are more balanced."*

Following the examination, Henry Honest offered, "We need to help the kidney." He said we should continue with the nutritional program Imani was now practicing. He also stated he wanted to attempt an Accu-power* session. Ed and the other two children decided to go on a New York excursion to pass the time during Imani's Accu-power session.

Imani and I were escorted to a small treatment room by Henry Honest and one of his assistants. Imani was asked to lay face down on a soft mat that was positioned on the floor. I knelt down beside her and gently stroked her face, back, and arms throughout the procedure. The technique involved the use of approximately 35 tiny needles. He strategically placed the needles into Imani's lower back and the back of her left arm. After about ten minutes, Master Honest removed the

---

* Accu-power is a procedure similar to Acupuncture that involves needles, heated leaves, and gentle pressure on various parts of the body.

needles and placed what looked like small pieces of spinach leaves and brown clay over the spots where the needles had previously been inserted. Next, the spinach-looking matter was lit with an incense stick. Each piece was kept in place until it was too hot for Imani to tolerate. Her little body was then swathed with cotton balls that had been dipped in rubbing alcohol. Imani cried frantically while kicking and screaming throughout the entire Accu-power session!

Retrospection is a powerful thing. I now deeply regret not being better prepared with a plan of action for Imani on that day. Upon reflection, I feel I should have allowed Henry Honest o demonstrate with the needles and heated greenery on me first. That way, Imani might have been more at ease for that scary new experience. I do firmly believe in the practice of Accu-power and the great benefits which are achieved through its use. However, I lament the fact that this particular encounter was such an unpleasant one for Imani. I recoil whenever I think back on that day.

During another visit to New York City, Henry Honest stated, "Don't be surprised if they offer Imani chemotherapy on the next visit to the hospital." I became terribly distraught over the thought of allowing anyone to put "poison" into my child's body. I pondered on stories of individuals who talked about losing hair and weight or becoming violently ill after being exposed to chemotherapy. The very idea of infusing our daughter's precious little body with chemotherapy sickened me. Henry Honest further cautioned, "If they give her chemotherapy, don't allow them to give her more than five rounds in very small doses." I made a mental note of this pertinent information for future reference.

October 7, 2002
Following our dinner tonight, Imani walked up behind me and asked, "Mom, why did I get this thing on my arm?" She continued on with, "How come I see other people eating the wrong things and they don't have lumps?" What do I say?

TWELVE

Chemotherapy

June 28, 2002
Is there anyone else out there whose life is as shitty as mine?

D<small>R</small>. S<small>ILVERCORE</small>* <small>WAS A WOMAN</small> who appeared to be in her early 30s and was a member of the oncology staff at the children's hospital. Tall and slender, she had an endearing mannerism that conveyed an individual who was totally committed to seeing children healthy and intact.

One particularly sunny, hazy, hot, and humid day, Dr. Silvercore called our home to recommend chemotherapy treatments for Imani.

The oncologist mentioned how Imani's type of cancer was so rare that she'd have to create a "special formula" of experimental chemotherapy. During that conversation, I felt severely harried! I'd heard and read dreadful stories about people who had received chemotherapy treatments. I envisioned Imani with all of her hair falling out while becoming emaciated due to the nausea and loss of appetite. For me, the gross visualizations were completely revolting.

---

* Name changed to protect her identity.

I called my mother that day and cried uncontrollably. I told her, "I don't want them to put poison into my baby's body!" My dear mother listened attentively. Then she offered in her familiar, maternal timbre, "If Imani needs chemotherapy in order to save her arm, let them give her a little bit."

Shortly after that, a meeting was set up for us to talk with Dr. Silvercore more extensively. I really don't remember the weather on that morning. *Was it Sunny? Cloudy? Raining?* I don't recall the trip north to the hospital that day. I can't even remember which conciliatory relative cared for my other two children. I was totally frozen with fear. I felt like I was in an abhorrent state of being. I was living a nightmare. Ed, Imani, and I exchanged nervous banter that morning.

When we arrived at the oncology unit, we were met by a social worker. She was a genial individual who explained some things about the program. I have very little recollection about what she shared. Her words were indecipherable to me due to my emotional, mental, and physical state that day. I managed an occasional smile and a head nod. Ed followed along and asked the questions during that session. As I glanced around the room, my heart sank. On the windowsill, there was a bronze statue of a man who appeared to be walking. The man bore a look of determination. Upon closer inspection, I noticed that the individual also had a prosthetic device for one leg. The creator of the figurine had artistically maneuvered the bronze material to display forward movement. It was a beautiful piece of artwork. Viewing the model sent chills up and down my spine.

There were other families in the waiting area of the oncology unit. I witnessed the faces of helpless fathers and despondent mothers. Fear was abundant in that place. There were children who looked weak and tired from the effects of their treatment. Some of the children were bald. Most had extremely pale skin and bloated faces. It was exceedingly upsetting to look into their eyes because I sensed their spirits were in need of relief. Tears began to fill my eyes. In that moment, it was clear to me that there are hundreds … no, thousands of families who face the unfathomable stress and strain of cancer each day!!!!

After a while, the social worker gave us a hand-made, crocheted, blue and lavender cap for Imani. She told us about a group of volunteers who knit the attractive hats for the children losing their hair as a result of the chemotherapy treatments. There was plenty of literature available to read and a delightful assortment of hats in a box on a nearby table. Some hats even had cute little braids under the rim that gave the appearance of hanging hair.

Imani was then escorted to a play area by a young, vibrant hospital assistant. There was an activity table stocked with construction paper, glue, scissors, crayons, paint, glitter, buttons, colorful feathers, decorative string, and lots of other hands-on materials. Another little person occupied the table where Imani chose to sit. The child wore a hospital gown and had a clear tube in her nostrils. Imani sat cautiously and began to create a masterpiece. The companionable assistant engaged both children in conversations about their artwork while I looked on sympathetically. It took every morsel of my sanity to keep me from running away from the hospital screaming like a maniac on that summer day!!!!!!

Finally, Dr. Silvercore came into the activity area. She greeted the little ladies at the table and winked at her proficient helpmate. Dr. Silvercore then beckoned for Ed and me to meet with her privately. My knees wobbled as I made the trek down the long corridor to her office. Once inside, Dr. Silvercore began asking a series of questions about Imani's general well-being. The doctor transcribed notes as we surrendered data regarding our daughter. After an uncomfortable pause, Dr. Silvercore declared, "I won't be able to offer any chemotherapy to Imani." A voice inside my head exploded with excitement,

"Is she saying what I think she's saying?" Dr. Silvercore explained that this cancer was such a rarity and that studies had shown the myxofibro sarcoma to be non-responsive to chemotherapy. She discussed the possibility of concocting a unique batch of chemicals for Imani, but ultimately confessed that given the exceptional circumstances regarding Imani's left arm, she was unsure about how to proceed in our case. I thought, *"Imani will NOT have to endure the horrors of chemotherapy? WHEW!"* Ed and I gazed at each other and did not speak for what seemed like several minutes. I don't know what he was thinking but, the voice inside my head now shrieked, ***"Hallelujah!!!"***

THIRTEEN

Where is the Love?

THE DAYS THAT FOLLOWED WERE both outlandish and consecrated. As the summer of 2002 came to a close, I became sickened by the prospect of returning to the classroom as a teacher of students with special needs. I explained to Ed that I didn't feel I was ready to fulfill my teaching responsibilities and he became furious. He failed to take into consideration the emotional duress I was facing each day. Every waking moment of my life centered on thoughts of Imani's well-being. I knew I desperately needed to spend time cocooning. The process of cocooning would allow me to pray, focus, and renew my spirit so I could function at my greatest level for the benefit of Imani's healing. This additional knowledge only further incensed Ed. He claimed I was an emotional wreck and insisted that I return to my classroom assignment at the designated time with my colleagues.

Two weeks before the commencement of that particular school year, I made an appointment with my building principal to share all that had transpired over that summer. She extended a sympathetic ear as well as a shoulder for me to cry on. My thoughtful principal directed me to the school district's human resource office and advised me to apply for the Family Medical Leave Act (FMLA). That way, she explained, I could spend 12 weeks at home replenishing my spirit while caring for Imani. At the conclusion of the 12 weeks, I would be guaranteed my teaching job.

One day during the 12 weeks of the approved FMLA period, Ed returned home in the middle of the day. He found me in the bathtub totally submerged in steamy bubbles and surrounded with several aromatic candles. The scornful look on his face was followed by his vile words, "Your ass needs to be at work. There's nothing wrong with you!" My heart sank.

Even with my parents' fulfilled promise to take responsibility for my portion of the household bills until I was able to return to work, Ed was vehement towards me. For the life of me, I couldn't convince Ed that it was imperative for me to spend extended time in prayer, meditation and proper preparation of meals (with tea and supplements). I desperately needed to be quiet and focused during that turbulent phase. Positive energy and optimistic thoughts were required as a way of promoting healing and health for Imani.

Conversely, Ed became more disconnected than ever before. He refused to talk to me. Ed had often used the lack of communication tactic in our 17+ years as husband and wife. He was one who would go days, weeks, and sometimes months without talking to me when he was upset. Ordinarily, his lack of interest in me crushed me at my core. However, his silent phase during the FMLA ordeal was the first time it didn't bother me at all. I was in a different place. Regardless of the devastating condition of my marriage, I was steadfast about being in a peaceful, productive space. I realized Imani needed me to exert my energy in unequivocal ways.

July 29, 2002
My left arm aches. I don't know if it's psychosomatic or if there's something wrong in there. It sometimes feels like

my left arm and left hand get a strange tingling sensation ... something like an uncomfortable cramp. H - E - L - P!

I need Ed to be the sole provider for the children today. I decided to spend the day with ME. My agenda:

> *got my hair done
> *had a pedicure
> *drove down to the beach
> *cried
> *did some reading (<u>Getting the Love you want</u> by Harvelle Hendrix)
> *cried
> *prayed
> *cried, cried, cried

Most of my thoughts are centered on Imani. I needed the day to regroup and rejuvenate . . . BREATHE (aaahhh)!

FOURTEEN

"I need a hamburger!"

**August 17, 2002**
My father called today. I know he could sense the emotional distress in my voice. He spoke with a calm assurance. I remember him saying, "It's going to be okay. I'm certain of it. This is something we just have to go through." I want to believe him.

ED AND I DECIDED TO try and help the children enjoy our trips to New York City whenever we visited the Natural Remedies Center. Following our time with Henry Honest, during one particular appointment, we went to Ground Zero, the previous location of the World Trade Center. I'm certain the children were unable to grasp the significance of that awesome site. However, I was overcome with a surreal sense of humility with each step I took.

Then, we were off on a ferryboat adventure to see the Statue of Liberty and Ellis Island. Our three children expressed their delight as they rode the ferryboat. They seemed to gain pleasure from the day's events and asked several questions about the historic displays on Ellis Island.

On the return trip from seeing Lady Liberty, we were all hungry. We decided to eat at Josie's, a vegetarian restaurant. Josie's is a great place with a wonderful menu for both adults and children. They feature salads and healthy drinks. They also have organic meats, healthy sweet potato fries, and delicious fruit smoothies. Josie's even has wholesome oatmeal-raisin cookies for dessert and pies made with organic ingredients.

By this time, we had been practicing a more "healthy" way of eating for more than a month. Each time we left the house, I carried along a small cooler stocked with foods from Imani's restricted diet. Most of the time, Imani appeared to be very unhappy whenever we traveled with that little red cooler. It was often filled with bottles of water, various cut-up fruit, an assortment of organic, whole grain breads or crackers, and a container with a healthy meal I had prepared the night before.

No matter what I lovingly prepared, Imani looked as if she was about to burst into tears at every mealtime setting. My heart ached for her throughout each meal. At the restaurant that day, I ate what Imani ate from the cooler while Ed and our other two children ordered from the menu. The truth of the matter was that I didn't really have much of an appetite anyway. I just wanted to see our child's health improve. I knew Imani didn't like the change in her diet, but I also knew it was imperative to stick to the strict regimen in order to evoke a positive change.

Everyone was fatigued upon our return to Delaware. It had been a busy day and I looked forward to a well-deserved rest. As we neared our home, I heard a small voice from the back seat. My outspoken, 12-year-old son said, "Dad, I need a hamburger!" The request surprised me not only because I thought all three children were asleep, but also because our family diet no longer consisted of hamburgers! No one spoke a word after that. There was an awkward silence throughout our family vehicle as Ed made an abrupt U-turn to the nearest fast food restaurant. The peculiar silence continued until Ed ordered, "Can I get a hamburger?" Ed handed the small bag to our son and headed toward home. Edwin removed his delicacy from the bag and began to devour the contents. The succulent aroma of that particular hamburger tantalized my taste buds and I began to salivate like one of Pavlov's dogs. Still, no one in the car spoke a word. The only sound came from Edwin's mouth as he consumed his tasty treat. I thought to myself, "Why couldn't he at least have waited until we got home to chow down in private instead of torturing the rest of us with those savory smells?"

In contemplation of that day, I now recognize how badly Edwin needed that hamburger. We were all totally stressed out at that point. We wanted relief from the horrendous nightmare that had become our lives. The burger represented the way life was before all of the fear, uncertainty, and doctor's visits. It was a reminder of a simpler time when daily living was not so traumatic. We **all** needed a hamburger! **We were all desperate for relief.**

August 27, 2002

Somehow, I convinced Ed to be present for a family meeting today. The five of us needed to express our feelings about everything that was happening. There was lots of crying. I'm glad the cleansing is evident. I know I feel much better when stuff isn't bottled up. Edwin is angry, Ebony is puzzled, and Imani is scared. Ed was silent. I know we're going to get through this. My foremost query is, "What will we look like when this battle is over?"

FIFTEEN

"Now, Faith..." (Hebrews 11:1)

<u>*February 28, 2003*</u>
I LOVE to hear them laughing. I feel so bad about the way the past year has affected all of us. We've all been emotionally damaged. It's time to heal. Today is another snow day. The children are playing outside in the snow with Ed and the dogs, Oreo & Bear. My heart warms at the sound of their joy.

As THE DOG DAYS OF summer passed and the leaves transformed their hues, I became more diligent than ever in my quest of health and healing for my family. During one phase of the process, I was overcome with emotion and bawled while telling myself, "If God wants to take Imani then I will give her back the way she was given to me ... with two arms!" In those moments of desperation, fear and faith traded places. I began to recognize that it was imperative to truly trust and believe in God in a manner that I had never done before.

Faith was ushered in like the mass choir at a church revival. I began to visualize Imani's left arm completely healed. With each new day, as fear and anxiety crept into my psyche, I began to praise God for Imani's life. Henry Honest taught us that we all have the power to heal ourselves. He further stated that it takes the body 270 days to heal itself. That new revelation astounded me as I reached for a red marker and my kitchen calendar to outline the route as a visual illustration of Imani's healing. During those nine months, the prayer on my lips shifted from, "Oh God, please heal Imani!" to "Thank you God for Imani's complete and total healing!"

Inevitably, fear acquiesced to the miraculous power of faith! The more I offered praise and thanks, the better I could discern the reality of having a child with **NO CANCER!!!**

All the while, my spirit was uplifted due to the incredible out-pouring of Love, Prayers, and Fasting with family, friends, and well-wishers. The following is an excerpt from an email that was sent on our behalf from a compassionate friend;

Subject: CALLING ALL WARRIORS OF LOVE!!!
ACTIVE DUTY REQUIRED - ALL WARRIORS OF LOVE !!!

MY DEAR FRIEND VIVIANE AND HER 8 YEAR OLD DAUGHTER, IMANI, ARE IN NEED OF YOUR INTERCESSION. IMANI HAS A GROWTH IN HER ARM WHICH WAS BIOPSIED IN MAY 2002. HER BONE AND CAT SCANS CAME BACK NEGATIVE...WHICH WAS GREAT NEWS...THERE WAS NO CANCER. IN JUNE 2002 (LAST MONTH), THE GROWTH HAD INCREASED. THE DOCTORS ARE SO CONCERNED ABOUT THE GROWTH THAT THEY SUGGESTED THE AGGRESSIVE SURGERY OF AMPUTATING MOST OF IMANI'S LEFT ARM.
THIS IS WHAT IMANI AND HER FAMILY NEED FROM YOU:

TO STORM HEAVEN AND EARTH WITH PRAYER, ENERGY, AND POWER. TO CALL ON THE UNIVERSE TO HEAL ONE OF ITS OWN. WHAT I CALL GOD OR JESUS, YOU MAY CALL, YAHWEH, JEHOVAH, ALLAH, BUDDHA, UNIVERSE, LOVE, ENERGY, THE WAY, THE LIGHT, SPIRIT...WHATEVER YOU CALL HER, HIM, IT... PLEASE CALL!!! AND CALL AGAIN AND AGAIN. I DON'T KNOW WHAT TOMORROW HOLDS, OR FOR THAT MATTER, EVEN LATER TODAY, BUT WHAT I KNOW FOR SURE IS THAT THE MYSTERY OF GOD AND THE UNIVERSE ARE AVAILABLE TO US WHEN WE COME TOGETHER IN COLLECTIVE LOVE !!! WE HAVE POWER ... PLEASE USE IT FOR IMANI TODAY. UNDERGIRD THEM WITH LOVE AND SEND THE POWER THEIR WAY!!! PLEASE SEND THIS TO EVERY PERSON YOU KNOW. I AM REQUESTING THAT THIS EMAIL GO ALL OVER THE WORLD AND THAT THE POWER OF GOD, THE UNIVERSE AND THE GALAXIES WILL BE UNLEASHED IN IMANI'S ARM AND BODY. I BELIEVE ... PLEASE BELIEVE WITH ME!!!

We continued with the healthy eating regimen while Imani was given the teas and supplements. I measured Imani's arm (circumference) weekly and kept a record of her weight.

MRI results from July 30, 2002
"There is extensive recurrent tumor, which has progressed since the previous study. It spans the humerus from the top of the shoulder for approximately 20cm in length. It involves the width of the upper arm, spanning approximately 8x8cm in diameter. It involves the deltoid muscle and extends behind the scapula. It infiltrates the muscles of the humerus with large degree of enhancing tumor. A large cystic region along the lateral

aspect of the humerus measures approximately 8x3x6 cm. The tumor surrounds the humeral shaft...

Impression: Extensive recurrent sarcoma of the left upper arm, progressed since April 2002."

Imani's arm measurements and weight (a)

Date	Left arm	Right arm	Weight
6/17/2002	26 cm	18.5 cm	58 lbs
7/11/2002	29 cm	18.5 cm	58 lbs
9/7/2002	25 cm	18.5 cm	58 lbs
9/21/2002	22.5 cm	18.5 cm	58 lbs

Dr. Portalmen and Dr. Silvercore recommended that Imani be retested every three months. At long last, the breakthrough we all so desperately needed came the day before Imani's ninth birthday. In September 2002, Imani's MRI report came back with the following information;

"The previously demonstrated tumor recurrence within the soft tissues of the left upper arm have markedly improved."

The report continued with:

"...on the prior MRI examination (the tumor) has diminished in size by at least fifty percent (50%). There is no evidence for extension into the shoulder joint. There are no other soft tissue masses demonstrated."

As a result, Imani's ninth birthday was celebrated in the spirit of awesome wonder!

September 27, 2002
Imani surprised me when I picked her up from school today. After struggling with her seatbelt for a few minutes, she looked up at me and smiled when she heard the familiar "click". Then she blurted out, "Mom, I'm a Healer". All I could manage to say in that moment of ecstasy was, "Yes, you are Beloved. Yes you are!"

Imani's arm measurements and weight (b)

Date	Left arm	Right arm	Weight
10/7/2002	23 cm	18.5 cm	58 lbs
10/12/2002	22.5 cm	18.5 cm	59 lbs
10/20/2002	22.5 cm	18.5 cm	58 lbs
11/16/2002	22 cm	18.5 cm	60 lbs
12/7/2002	21.5 cm	18.5 cm	60 lbs

December 27, 2002
The hospital called. Imani's CAT scan revealed NO mass in her lungs or chest!

"I will praise you Lord, with all my heart. I will tell of all the marvelous things you have done" (Psalm 9:1).

January 24, 2003
Today marks the six month point for our journey with the Japanese teas. (Whew!)

Imani had an MRI appointment at the hospital. The technicians were amazed at her progress. They couldn't figure out which arm they were supposed to examine. They laughed out loud when Imani assured them it is the arm with the scar. It's hard to see the difference in the sizes of her arms because there's been such visual progress. On Monday, I hope to get the results from our pediatrician. The waiting is torturous!!!

I've got to calm my Spirit.

March 15, 2003
Imani is doing remarkably well. She's still on the tea and taking daily supplements. We still have to watch what she eats. Her left arm is (some swelling) slightly bigger than her right arm. I get nervous every time Imani tells me she doesn't feel well. I literally have to talk myself out of a state of panic whenever she mentions she has a headache. I'm learning that I have to walk in the Faith that Imani is healed for the rest of my life.

Imani's arm measurements and weight (c)

Date	Left arm	Right arm	Weight
1/17/2003	20.5 cm	18.5 cm	60 lbs
2/11/2003	20.5 cm	18.5 cm	60 lbs
2/28/2003	20 cm	18.5 cm	60 lbs
4/25/2003	21 cm	18.5 cm	63 lbs
5/2/2006	18.5 cm	17 cm	

April 21, 2003
We just returned from New York. Henry Honest put Imani on something he calls "graduation tea". He says she is clearly 90-99% better. From our first meeting,

I remember him saying, "It takes the body 270 days to heal itself". That means it takes about nine months for the body to complete the cycle of healing. That now makes so much sense to me! It's been nine months and Imani is HEALED! There are no words to describe the relief and joy I am experiencing!!!

Fast Forward…

The MRI report from February 9, 2006 announced:

"Clinical history is tumor…
No evidence for mass or soft tissue swelling. The muscles are in normal limits. The humerus is normal.
Impression: Post surgical scarring of left upper arm. No evidence for mass or other acute abnormality."

<u>February 9, 2007</u>
The doctor called today. He said Imani's MRI report came back with no traces of cancer! It's been five years now. So much has happened … Whew!!! I'm so grateful for Imani's left arm. So thankful for her life. This journey has been miraculous!!!!!

Our lovely, healthy Imani was fifteen years old when the final MRI was conducted on November 25, 2008.

The medical report states:

"There is no evidence of significant marrow abnormality of the humerus. Slight fatty replacement of the lateral musculature of the upper arm is noted. There is no evidence of any measurable

soft tissue mass or drainable fluid collection nor is there significant edema or mass in the intrinsic muscle bundles. The humerus shows no significant marrow abnormality.

Impression: There does not appear to be any suspicious bone or soft tissue abnormality of the left upper arm."

ALL PRAISES, ALL PRAISES!!!

Epilogue

*"And now abide faith, hope, **love**, these
three; but the greatest of these is **love**."*

(I CORINTHIANS 13:13)

A LOVE BEYOND THE REALM of comprehension healed Imani. I am learning to live into the gift of healing as a daily exercise. I begin each day in the spirit of gratitude and amazement. To date, I have been blessed with opportunities to provide an oral account of this mind-blowing saga. I have received a wide range of feedback. A few of the varied comments have been;

"Your daughter never had cancer."
"I would have been leery about that Japanese Healer."
"You guys got lucky!"

Nevertheless, my reply is grounded in **Love**. My faith walk fashioned my response to the comments above. *"Imani is 22 years old with two arms and no cancer!"* **Love** trumps everything!

It was agape **love** that comforted me as I trusted God and let go of an unhealthy marriage in 2004. Abiding **love** anchored me as I obtained a Doctorate degree in Educational Leadership on May 19, 2013.

God's miraculous **love** sustains Imani daily. She is a 2015 graduate of Delaware State University with a Bachelor of Science degree in Public Health. Ironically, Imani was a student ambassador for the Thurgood Marshall program on campus and also volunteered with a program for cancer research. **Love** overpowers me with awe and wonder each time I look at the scar on my youngest child's left arm. **Love** left a significant mark. The scar tissue on Imani's left arm is stronger than the original flesh ever was. She is a living testament to the fact that miracles can and do still happen.

Endearing **love** covers Ebony. She is a 2014 graduate of Howard University with a Bachelor's degree in Business Marketing. Currently, Ebony is a Leader in the Apparel department at the Nike Community Store in Washington, DC. At 23 years old, Ebony is also actively in pursuit of a Master's degree in Project Management. I marvel at her ability to focus on tasks and her tenacious personality.

"The Lord gave and the Lord has taken away. Blessed be the name of the Lord."

JOB 1:21

Eternal **love** personifies Edwin. On July 6, 2014, my beloved son died in a motorcycle accident. There are no words to adequately describe the anguish of losing my handsome Chocolate Prince. Fortunately, I was blessed to spend quality time with him a few hours before he mounted his bike for that final ride. Our very last goodbye included a tender embrace as Edwin leaned over me with those muscular arms and shoulders. What followed was a warm kiss on my cheek from his thick, full lips as Edwin avowed, "I **love** you Mom."

Although I face days of unmanageable sadness, I'm elated that Edwin read the manuscript to <u>Armor of Faith …A mother's memoir</u> a few years ago and gave me an enthusiastic stamp of approval. My son was excited that I was able to record our experiences to share with others. He mentioned remembering that time in our lives from a child's perspective and that he was grateful to be able to glean a more mature understanding of what was going on as an adult. I am delighted that he further offered his artistic skills by drawing the cover for this publication. I experience a happy-sorrow whenever I recall Edwin exclaiming, "Mom, we've got to get this story out!" On Mother's Day 2009, Edwin presented me with a poster he had created with the following message:

FAITH = F–ocus
A–nd
IT
H–appens

My son recognized that focusing is imperative in order to achieve desired outcomes. Edwin came to understand that miraculous things can happen when you adjust your focus, change your mind, and change your diet. The ability to focus was an essential component of this journey. The need to focus was crucial in order for us to arrive at this sacred place.

The holy scriptures exhort us to visualize "a cloud of witnesses" (Hebrews 12:1) that provide encouragement as we face challenges in this life. I imagine my heavenly ancestors consoling me. My heart rejoices as I envision my fine-looking, dark, muscular, artistic, intelligent, loving, humorous son, as the leader of my spiritual cheering squad chanting for me and supporting my efforts to advance on this life-journey, no matter the tests or trials that confront me! I believe

Edwin knew that this **love** story would help somebody to experience Faith in an empowering, inspiring and transforming manner. I know God's **love** will lead, comfort and sustain you in the same manner it has me. In the end, **love** conquers all.

May 4, 2003
Another dream...

Imani was playing kickball outside with a group of friends. She stood confidently at first base. I ran over to her to help her tag someone out. As I ran closer, I screamed, "Tag them out, Imani!!!" At the last possible moment, Imani caught the ball and casually touched the base with her foot. Then she looked over at me and smiled. In that instance, I heard a soft, reassuring voice say, "Imani will be alright without you."

Copy of Letter regarding amputation of Imani's left arm

Division *of* Oncology

November 6, 2002

RE:
MRN:
DOB: 09/28/93
DOV: 11/01/02

Dear Dr.

I had the pleasure of seeing   in followup at the
As you know,   was first seen in May of this year for a left arm mass that had been growing since February of 2002. The biopsy was originally read as a benign myxoma but, on review, the tissue was felt to be more consistent with a malignant myxofibrosarcoma. The pathology had been sent to several other institutions for review. Our recommendation to the family has been amputation of the left arm as this type of sarcoma is unresponsive to chemotherapy. The family chose to obtain a second opinion and monitor   and, since last seen in August of 2002, she has been seen by a homeopathic healer. She has had dietary changes where she has been eating a lot of whole grains and raw fruits and vegetables. Additionally, she has been taking Japanese teas, sea weeds, aloe vera and several other herbal remedies. In that time, the parents have noted that the arm circumference has decreased from 31 cm to 22.5 cm. They have been measuring it at the largest area. As well, she had a repeat MRI of the arm at the end of September which also showed a decrease in size of the mass. There does not appear to be any invasion into the lymph glands, nor has there been any invasion into the chest wall.

On evaluation today,   is well appearing. She does have, on her HEENT examination, several small mobile anterior cervical and possibly supraclavicular, nodes. None of these measure more than 0.5 cm. She has no axillary lymphadenopathy and no inguinal lymphadenopathy. Her left arm, although clearly with a greater circumference than the right arm, has decreased in size overall. There was a cystic component at her last visit that is now not palpable. Her exam is otherwise normal.

In summary,   is a nine year old with a possible myxofibrosarcoma that appears to be regressing. There has been some controversy as to the histology of this tumor and, if it is regressing, it is highly unlikely that it is a sarcoma. I am very pleased that with no intervention the tumor is decreasing in size and agree with the family's plan to continue to monitor it. I have no objections to the herbal remedies that they are receiving, especially if they have made a difference in the overall outcome. I would like her to have an evaluation done to make sure that

the tumor has not spread. I have given the family a prescription today for a neck and chest CT. She should continue to get MRI scans of that arm every three months and we would like to see her back in February of next year.

Please feel free to contact us with any questions or concerns.

Sincerely,

Interview with Henry Honest

The following conversation between Viviane Philmon (**VP**) and Henry Honest (**HH**) took place in New York City on October 11, 2006.

VP: How long have you been teaching people to heal themselves?

HH: Probably over 50 years.

VP: Is there a vast difference in working with children as opposed to working with adults?

HH: Yes. Children are easy for me because they are more pure than adults. Adults have so many experiences. They are also stressed and many, many things. With children, the problem is no knowledge; no experience. That's why it's good for me; Pure, easy to reach the consciousness of organs; the system. That's why children are easy. The problem with my herbal teas and also supplements is the kind of taste. We don't put any sugar in it. We don't manipulate it. It's done. It's a pure taste. So children have a problem drinking the tea or taking the supplements. But if the mother is clever enough, she will put juice or honey or jelly or fruit drink into the tea. Most children who have a consciousness to cure themselves, they don't care. They will drink it. Amazing!

VP: What was your initial impression of Imani when you met her?

HH: I connected with her organs; each organ. Everything was beautiful but I felt her digestion meridian system was broken. I asked (her body) if this was cancerous or cancer or an infection. I didn't tell the mother or family because this is a pretty severe medical report and I have to respect that. So, I talked with her body and her body said to me it's really an infection the body made more than cancer cells. That's why I said, I asked her, "How are your bowel movements?" and she said, "Well, I don't go enough." And the mother said to me, "Yeah. Well, we go to the doctor." The doctor said things more seriously. For me, it was very serious. We just needed to clean up the colon. That's why I gave her time to cure the constipation. Also, the infection was more than cancer. Mostly, I try to cure imbalances. That was my concern because I connect with each organ system's consciousness. They (body systems) know what they have to do. Unfortunately, many things can get to the liver to stop the function and make the liver weak. Then it can't break a tumor or can't break cancer, you know. So the bacteria to the weak part will make cancer grow more. Her situation is really, really more than anything, the infection – especially constipation is spoiled and more bacteria will overgrow. So it interfered with the large intestine meridian so her arm is growing up more; got bigger.

VP: Can you talk a bit about the teas and supplements that were given to Imani during the summer of 2002?

HH: Yeah. My consciousness told me what her body wanted. The overgrown bacteria virus – her body said, "I want to kick them out." That's why the supplements and teas are designed to break down blockages. So I made up from Nature things like a Grandfather or Grandmother…Wisdom. Then I gave her a combination of natural herbs for breaking down bad blockage and a little breaking down of good blockage too. There must be a balance. Then, totally I want to make the communication well between the brain through the spine to the body. Body information then going from the spine to the brain. Then I want to go one hundred percent with information from the brain to the spine.

VP: Is there ever a time that you consult with client's doctors regarding their medical condition?

HH: Actually, I respect doctors very much. Because he found Imani's problem, he is due respect. More than respect, I just want to follow what her body wants. The important thing is more than controlling the patient or curing the symptom. I need to get to the core of this. She is young. She has a long life (ahead). If we cure only the symptom and not get to the core, maybe she will make it (the lump) again. So my concern is asking her body, "What is the cause of this?" If all great, clever doctors would begin to think about the core, this would be wonderful! Many, many doctors call me to introduce their patients and I help them because they find the symptom and I need to teach what the causes are. Yes.

VP: When you shared information with us about the possible need for small amounts of chemotherapy being used to treat Imani, I have to admit that I was disturbed. You

will recall that you warned us about the hospital probably
offering the chemotherapy. How do you now explain your
approach at that time given the fact that you initially told
us Imani did NOT have cancer?

HH: The cancer pulse inside of the organs communicates
as something very weak. It has kind of a "nothing" reaction.
Her reaction (pulse) is like a Discothèque. My experience has
been that her pulse showed an infection. If it is cancer, the
body freaks out. The pulse is going to be like nothing. But
her pulse is very exciting. Also, if it is really cancer, the liver
functioning is really weak. The liver blood goes to the small
intestine to help the digestive system. If her pulse is like weak
– very no power – no pressure – it shows cancer. Cancer, I
feel is a more ugly tumor. Her tumor part did not show pain.
Cancer shows a shut down connection. Her body part (the
left arm) still showed a connection with her. That's why I felt
this is more than cancer. She was fighting against an infection. Sure, it was a cancerous infection but, not really cancer.
That's what I felt anyway. Also, the cancer smell is a little different. The infection smells and cancer smells are different.
It's very hard to explain. This is from my experience.

VP: I'm certain that you are aware that medical insurance
companies do not accept alternative therapy as a viable
treatment for cancer. Therefore, families have to pay out of
pocket if they seek to go this route for healing. Personally
speaking, I know that it can be a financial strain on a family at such a critical time. However, I must note that you
NEVER once put pressure on our family to pay you for
services even when we were (at times) thousands of dollars
in debt to you. What made you decide to continue with

Imani's treatments when we were so far behind in paying you for the teas, supplements and expertise?

HH: I don't know what you are meaning – what you are asking me but my concern; the important thing was Imani. Her recovery was most important. Money is an exchange for services. I am originally a Healing Minister. So, the money is an appreciation to our knowledge – our experiences. Free money doesn't work. I have helped thousands of people without charging. They complain about the taste. They complain, "I can't take this today." They call and say, "My house is smelling bad!" Or, "This is a ridiculous taste!" Many people complain. They have to really concentrate. That's very hard for somebody who doesn't have enough money. But I think I better charge them because then they are more serious. If it were free, they don't take it serious. That's no good. That's why, unfortunately, we need some kind of limit. I have worked with thousands of people without charging many times and my record was very bad; ten percent or nine percent recovered. The others just complained. They did not appreciate my gifts. That's why I decided with you, you're not poor but, you're not rich enough. I needed to do as much as I can; less – then we had to respond to each other. Then when you had money sometimes, you pay little by little. Pay enough and that's okay. I knew when I met you that you were desperate to see your daughter well. I know you would send the money so I never worried about that. I knew you would appreciate what I do (my ministry). The money was not to pay for me. You pay for yourself through appreciation. That's how we do. Mostly in my Japan, in our clinic, we don't charge you. You bring a potato or a cucumber or rice, you know. And then it's okay. That's my original thinking. Yeah.

VP: What message would you like to share with others who may be facing a similar situation involving their child?

HH: Okay. The child is fortunately very pure. They have less toxins than us. Our body is a Spiritual foundation. I want to send positive energy to the Spirit, Mind and Body. Our center is a bridge of consciousness. When our body is in harmony, we don't get sick. Children have a beautiful inner Spiritual foundation. Their consciousness is good. Unfortunately, we feed it fancy food, sweets and things that make us struggle. Yeah. Even our animals – we feed them and make their immune system weak. But wild animals are different. They don't get sick. If we give children pure food, they will be fine. I even recommend meat. You can eat it. You can eat a little bit – not a lot. That's the key. Balance and pure. As long as we give them (children) a great Spiritual foundation continuously, Physical foundation and Consciousness, Love, Respect and Caring. Then teach them to be proud. The organs know what they have to do. But if you give them bad food or a bad consciousness/actions, then they cannot be pure. If children follow their nature, they will be very successful. That will prevent sickness.

VP: Will you share some of your plans for the near future?

HH: My plan is the safe food. I want to make a medicine food; just a healthy food.

Also, I will include the combination of exercise – not Sports! I will teach Do–In–Koh exercise, Tai–Chi, and Yoga or some life spiritual exercise. As long as we respect each other and love each other; take care of each other, I think we won't need so many drugs. Maybe drug companies will find this is a great thing. Then we can improve each other.

VP: Henry Honest, please know our family is eternally grateful to you for all you've done and continue to do for us. We thank you so much for everything. We applaud you and extend blessings and peace to you in all of your future endeavors!

HH: You are quite welcome. The important thing is that life is so beautiful. But if you are not in tune with your consciousness, you will not think beautifully. That's no good because some people think being yourself is bad. Most people lose their health and are unhappy because they don't do what they want to do...they don't! They also don't do what they want to be. They don't live the life they truly want to live. They fake it for the money or for some reputation...I don't know! They are losing who they are. Another important thing is learning. If you see a beautiful thing and you've never done it in your life; try it! Don't say, "I'm a woman". Or, "I'm over thirty". No excuses. Don't say, "I don't have that kind of money". No! Just take chances! That means you are really 15-20 years younger than you really are. That means you receive incredible, pure joy and creativity and artistic ability! If I don't like it, I can say, "I'm sorry, I can't take it". If I don't know, I say, "I'm sorry, I don't know". That's the key. People should say, "Maybe I **can** make it". Say, "Yes...I will!" You've got to be flexible. We need it. Yes.

VP: Again, I Thank you.

HH: You are quite welcome.

(Smiles and hugs)

Recipes

THE FOLLOWING RECIPES ARE SUGGESTIONS for individuals who are attempting to transform their eating habits to a more holistic way of living. Keep in mind that Imani's diet was quite restricted due to her diagnosis. At the time, the decision was made to convert our entire family to foods that are made of pure ingredients (no pesticides, no preservatives, no dyes, NO MSG) while including more water and more raw fruits and vegetables. My personal goal was to make sure the meals I prepared were tasty and satisfying. I have found that the key was in the seasonings from the herbs and spices. Natural herbs like tarragon, lemon grass, coriander, cumin, turmeric, cinnamon, dill weed, and curry (just to name a few) truly enhance the flavor of foods. My suggestion is to visit your nearest health food store and try a new herb every week. You will be pleasantly surprised by the reaction of your family members. It is also a good idea to become acquainted with the whole foods magazines that are available. These magazines have many great suggestions for families who are striving to transition to a more healthy lifestyle. Finally, please be aware that while most of my meals were absolutely delicious, there were times that we had to resort to a meal consisting of almond butter and raw honey on organic wheat bread when the dinner was a total mishap. Don't be discouraged. Don't give up! All of the meals may not turn out the way you planned. Remember that it is all a learning process. Don't be afraid to be creative. Whenever I come across a new recipe, I always modify it to fit my family's needs. You know the people you are cooking for better than anyone else. So, make changes whenever you deem it necessary. Overall, it is important that you enjoy the experience!

<u>Helpful hints:</u>

The following items are included as things to keep in your kitchen as you embark on a new way of eating.

Extra virgin olive oil	Coriander	Black pepper
Organic butter	Bay leaves	Sea salt
Non-aluminum pots/pans	Vegetable broth	Raw sugar
Distilled water	Organic dried oregano	Unbleached flour
Fresh garlic cloves	Sage leaves	Cast iron skillet
Curry powder	Ground cumin	Wooden spoons
Raw honey	Fresh ginger root	
Organic apple cider vinegar	White/red/yellow onions	

Also, remember to have a wholesome variety of fresh fruits and vegetables in stock at all times! Be sure to include **beans** and **nuts** with your diet. Beans and nuts are a great source of proteins that are necessary as you work towards your optimum health. Here are a few examples that I have found to be delightful. Prepare the beans as the package directs. Then add quinoa (prepare as package instructs) and vegetables your family enjoys. Practice exercising creativity in your kitchen.

The nuts should be eaten as a healthy snack throughout the day. Be sure to avoid nuts with added salt and sugars. Organic, dry nuts are a tasty treat you and your children will learn to enjoy.

Beans	**Nuts**
Baby lima beans	Almonds
Lentil beans	Peanuts
Kidney beans	Walnuts
Black-eyed peas	Pumpkin seeds
Black beans	Sunflower seeds

Shrimp and Pasta Delight

2 c. fresh shrimp	1 box frozen green peas
organic angel hair pasta	1-2 tbs. Virgin olive oil
1 medium onion (chopped)	1-2 garlic cloves
1 tsp. Salt	1 tsp. Pepper
2 tsp. Lemon pepper	½ tsp. Tarragon (optional)

In a large colander, steam green peas for about 15 – 20 minutes. While peas are thawing, begin to cook pasta. Pasta should be prepared as directed from box.

Saute onions with garlic and olive oil in large skillet. Add shrimp and season with salt and peppers. Coat evenly and slowly add green peas. Mix well.

Place pasta in large bowl. Top with shrimp and peas. Sprinkle with tarragon.

Serve with fresh organic sliced tomatoes.

Enjoy ☺

Jan's Slam'n Slaw (Cole Slaw)

3 large Granny Smith apples   ½ head fresh organic cabbage
organic safflower mayonnaise   ½ tsp. fresh lemon juice

Optional:

1 cup dark brown or golden raisins
¼ cup crushed walnuts
¼ tsp. Celery seeds
1/8 tsp. Raw sugar

Preparation:

Cut up apples into chunks (discard seeds and apple cores)
Shred cabbage
Carefully mix all ingredients in a large bowl
Add safflower mayonnaise (to your personal preference)
Increase or decrease the amounts of the optional ingredients as you wish. Allow your taste buds to be your guide ☺

Substitution:

You may want to use some type of organic Caesar salad dressing in place of the safflower mayonnaise.

Refrigerate for one hour.
Serve as a side dish or afternoon/evening snack.

Black Bean Lasagna

2 cans of organic black beans

12 oz. organic ricotta cheese

1 box of organic lasagna noodles (uncooked)

1 tsp. Sea salt

½ tsp. White pepper

¼ tsp. Cumin

2 tbsp. Organic virgin olive oil

16 oz. Mild organic salsa

1 organic brown egg

½ tsp. Black pepper

¼ tsp. Coriander

1 medium white onion

Optional:

2 cups organic shredded cheese (cheddar)

1 lb. Organic ground turkey or beef

1 cup frozen corn

With wooden spoon, mix ricotta cheese and brown egg until smooth. Add seasonings and set aside.

In colander, drain all liquids from black beans. Rinse thoroughly. Gently mash black beans with a fork. Add salsa and mix thoroughly. (If you desire to use the meat and corn, now is the time to include these ingredients. Pour olive oil into hot skillet and sauté onion. Add meat and brown to your liking. Add the frozen corn when meat has browned sufficiently. Pour off any excess liquid).

Lightly grease the bottom and sides of a large lasagna container (preferably glass).

Begin layering container in the following manner;
Lasagna noodles, ricotta mixture, black bean mixture, shredded cheese, etc.

Be sure to end with the shredded cheese. Cover and bake at 350 degrees for one hour. Let cool for approximately 20 minutes before serving.

Serve with a garden salad. Include fresh spinach leaves to give your salad an extra appeal!

Fried Cabbage with Brown Rice (or Couscous)

1 medium head of cabbage	2 cups of organic brown rice
1 small white onion	1 cup green peppers (chopped)
1 cup red peppers (chopped)	1 cup yellow peppers (chopped)
½ cup of celery (chopped)	2 bay leaves
2 cups of water	2 cups of organic vegetable broth
2-3 tbsp. Virgin olive oil	1 tsp. Salt
½ tsp. Black pepper	½ tsp. White pepper
¼ tsp. Cumin	1-2 tsp. Tarragon (optional)

Preparation:

Cook brown rice/couscous according to directions on package. (Suggestion; Try substituting the vegetable broth for ½ of the amount of water you typically use for more flavorful rice/couscous. Also, add the bay leaves to the pot while waiting for the liquid to boil before adding brown rice/couscous).

Coarsely chop cabbage and place in colander. Rinse thoroughly with cool water. Let cabbage drain.

In large skillet, add olive oil and allow it to get very hot. Add chopped onion and celery and stir carefully about 1-2 minutes. Turn skillet down to a medium/low heat.

Use wooden spoon as you carefully add cabbage to skillet. Stir continuously. Now add peppers and seasonings. Keep stirring to coat all ingredients.

Place lid on top and simmer on low setting for 5 – 10 minutes. Sprinkle with Tarragon.

Place prepared rice/couscous in a large decorative serving bowl. Top with cabbage solution.

Serve with sliced and seeded organic apples and pears.

YUM!

Butter Bean Chili

1 lb. organic ground turkey (optional)
1 cup chopped onion
2 cloves garlic
1 16 oz. can tomatoes (stewed)
1 16 oz. can butter beans (drained)
1 8 oz. can tomato sauce
2 chopped seasonal peppers
(red, green or yellow)

1 tbsp. chili powder
½ tsp. organic brown sugar
1/8 tsp. ground red pepper
½ tsp. salt
½ tsp. dried basil (crushed)
¼ tsp. black pepper

Using a cast iron skillet, brown the meat with the onions, garlic, and peppers. Add all other ingredients and mix well. Bring mixture to boil. Reduce heat. Cover and simmer for 30 minutes.

Serve with brown rice (or couscous) and corn bread.

Stewed Apples

4 large Granny Smith apples
1-2 tsp. Cinnamon
½ tsp. Ground cloves
1 tsp. Organic raw sugar

4 medium red apples
½ tsp. Nutmeg
¼ tsp. Cardamom
1 tbsp. water

Preparation:
Remove skin and seeds from all apples. Slice apples (medium to thin width) and place into large mixing bowl. Add cinnamon, nutmeg, and ground cloves. Stir carefully to coat all apple slices. Add raw sugar and cardamom to apples and mix thoroughly.

Preheat oven to 350 degrees. Pour water into bottom of baking container. Add apples and top with lid. Bake apples for approximately 45 minutes (or until they are tender). Let apples cool for 10 minutes before serving. Delicious!!
Note: This same recipe is great using peaches and/or pears.

Enjoy!

About the Author

VIVIANE M. PHILMON WAS BORN in Philadelphia, Pennsylvania. She proudly wears the title of mother, daughter, sister, friend, educator, caregiver, singer, dancer, dreamer, and writer. Viviane has always had an interest in healthy living, fitness, and nutrition. She holds a Bachelor of Science Degree in Special Education from Indiana University of Pennsylvania, a Master's Degree in Curriculum and Instruction, and a Doctorate in Educational Leadership from Delaware State University. Her commitment to optimal health and her passion for children prompted her to write <u>Armor of Faith ... A Mother's Memoir.</u> She anticipates that the book will prove to be a catalyst for all who read it to make positive changes in their daily lives. Dr. Viviane Philmon currently resides in Dover, Delaware.